# Super Sperm Your Guy and Beat Infertility: The Ultimate Male Fertility Preparation Program

Other Books by the Author:

Dancing Your Way to Fertility
The Infertility Diaries
Your Daily Fertility Success Journal

Visit Amazon.com to learn more!

Super Sperm Your Guy and Beat Infertility: The Ultimate Male Fertility Preparation Program!

Paula Fuoco Davis

PaulaMediaandEntertainment.com, Nashua, NH

ISBN: 9781544703206

Edition Notice

Date of Publication

Number of Printings: First printing

Year of publication: 2016

Books may be purchased by contacting the publisher and author at:
Books may be purchased in quantity and/or special sales by contacting
the publisher, PaulaMediaandEntertainment.com or by email at
Frably@aol.com.


Books may be purchased in quantity and/or special sales by contacting
the publisher,

Library of Congress Catalog Number:
ISBN:
   1.  Infertility 2. Fertility 3. Health

     First Edition

This book is dedicated to the men in my journey, Christopher Davis, my husband, Joseph Fuoco, my father and my son, Sammy Brandon Davis. You all have made my journey complete and wonderful. Thank you for all the dedication, sacrifices and love you have given me.

Table of Contents

Paula Fuoco Davis: has been a newspaper reporter and journalist for the past 30 years. She has worked at The Lawrence Eagle-Tribune, The Nashua Telegraph and New Hampshire. She covered education, social issues and other feature stories. She founded and is editor of Commitment.com, an online site for women and authored more than 25 books. She is a survivor of infertility and wants others to have every single bit of information she didn't have. She has loved writing this book.

# Super Sperm Your Guy

Do you want your guy to have healthy sperm? What impact does your man's reproductive health have on your ability to get pregnant? This book is designed to help you help your guy be fertile and healthy.

Don't panic if your guy was diagnosed with a low sperm count. Just as there are many things a woman can do to maximize her fertility, there are also many things a man can do to improve the quality, quantity, and speed of his sperm.

Whether or not your guy was diagnosed with any specific problem, it is important to address his fertility because underlying, undiagnosed problems could exist in your man's reproductive system that are not being caught.

Some causes of inadequate sperm production include hormone imbalances, post-testicular issues with plumping or ejaculation, trauma or accidents, varicocele, or dilated veins in the scrotum, undescended testis/testes, excessive xenoestrogen, which are environmental estrogen exposure; infectious disease of the epidydimis, a diseased endocrine (glandular) system affecting the hypothalamus, pituitary, thyroid, adrenals and the testes, resulting in low DHEA and testosterone levels, congenital abnormalities, urethral stricture, malnutrition, especially protein deficiency.

It can sometimes take two to three months to improve the quality of sperm, so you'll want to begin preparing as soon as possible.

# Tests For Men

## Here are some of the tests your husband/partner can request:

• Sperm analysis, including a sperm antibody test, which can determine sperm count, motility, morphology (shape), seminal fluid, volume of ejaculation, and pH level.

• A Hormone Analysis: Hormones include testosterone, follicle stimulating hormone, and lutinizeing hormone which are critical to sperm production.

You may also want to have analyzed prolacin levels, thyroid stimulating hormone, sand ex-hormone binding globulin.

• Scrotal Doppler Ultrasound: measures the size of the testicle and look for blockages that involve transport of sperm out of the testicle.

• Transrectal Ultrasound: ultrasound technology is used to image the reproductive tract.

• A blood test to check for infections and hormone levels.

• A white blood cell count to detect infection, past infection, inflammation, low levels of inhibin B, or the compound alpha-glucosidase.

• Forward progression: this test measures the amount of forward movement in the sperm.

• Kruger morphology: if an abnormal morphology is found, this test allows the specialists to examine the sperm structure in great detail.

• Anti-sperm antibodies: this means the male has created an immunological response toward the sperm cells

• Sperm agglutination: sperm is examined to see whether there is any clumping together of the cells. Sperm agglutination can indicate the presence of sperm antibodies or bacterial infection.

• Viability: this test is performed if the sperm analysis shows that less than 30 percent of the sperm are motile. This test determines whether or not there is a presence of live sperm.

• Fructose: this test determines whether there is a blockage or no sperm at all being produced.

• An often overlooked cause of infertility in men is low-grade infection in the male urinary tract. Symptoms are often subtle and hard to diagnose, but they can include chills, fever, increased urination and intense burning during urination. Some physicians recommend culturing a semen sample to detect this mild infection.

# Cleanses To Boost His Fertility Potential

Here are some cleanses for men to consider before beginning infertility treatments.

• **A Parasite Cleanse:** Parasites can weaken sperm on a very hard-to-detect level. Health food stores carry 30-day parasite cleanses that can effectively remove parasites from the body.

• **Heavy Metal Cleanse:** Chemicals, pesticides and toxins in our environment have greatly impacted male fertility. Many men suffer from low-quality sperm because of these environmental toxins and chemicals. If possible, consider a heavy metal cleanse that can help remove these chemicals.

• **Liver Cleanse:** Just as detoxifying the liver is key to healing female infertility, it is equally important for men. Consider having your partner do a liver cleanse. The liver helps to filter toxins from the body, including excess hormones.

• **Candida-Yeast Cleanse:** can help rid the body of toxins.

• **Colon Hydrotherapy:** A colon cleanse can eradicate years of toxins in the large intestine, reducing the burden on the liver, pancreas, gall bladder and kidney.

## Holistic and Alternative Health Treatments to Consider

• **Acupuncture:** Acupuncture has been known to help men who have a low sperm count. It may be helpful for your partner to begin weekly or twice-weekly acupuncture treatments.

Make sure to let the acupuncturist know that you are looking to strengthen your husband's sperm Acupuncture points can help redirect Qi (energy) to key points in the body that assist in the smooth flow of blood to the penis and scrotum.

## • Bio Cleanse

An ionic food bath, also known as a bio cleanse ionic detox foot bath, pulls toxins out of the body through the feet. Positive and negative ions are emitted by the ionic foot bath machine, and helps the body rebalance and eliminate toxins in the kidneys, bowel, liver and skin.

A holistic practitioner in your area may have this machine that can remove yeast, parasites, and heavy metals from your liver, kidneys and muscles.

This should only be done as a preparation for infertility treatments, and not once you have started infertility medication or treatments, such as an IUI or IVF. It is not considered safe for anyone with an organ transplant, pacemaker or epilepsy.

## • Lymphatic Massage or Manual Lymphatic Drainage

This is a gentle massage that encourages the natural drainage of the lymph from the tissues in the body. This type of massage is very helpful to the lymph system and is an excellent way to detoxify. Stimulating the lymphatic system helps to drain swollen tissues, enhances the body's immune system, and helps the body's natural waste removal system.

## • Applied Kinesiology

In applied kinesiology, a chiropractor or holistic practitioner will use what is referred to a "the gun" or activator to release trauma and emotional pain in your body.

## • Craniosacral therapy

CranioSacral Therapy is a gentle, hands-on form of body work that releases tension in the layer of tissue called the fascia which surrounds the organs and nervous system. Craniosacral practitioners use light pressure on the skull and lower back to release restrictions on the body's craniosacral system. It is sometimes also done by massage therapists, naturopaths, chiropractors and others who work with the spine, skull and fascia to treat the body's central nervous system. Cranio-sacral can be a powerful tool in releasing past emotional and physical traumas. It can also improve hormone balance and blood flow, and help balance the spinal fluid and nervous system.

## • Blood Type Diet

The body has a chemical reaction to the foods you eat, and some holistic practitioners feel there is some benefit to eating in a way that is compatible with your blood type.

If you cannot follow this diet completely, it may help to just be aware of your blood type and take note if you feel more or less energized when you eat foods according to blood type.

There are many books available on eating for your blood type.

# • Homeopathy

Homeopathy is a great way to release and unblock emotional traumas or negative patterns that may be affecting your guy's fertility. Homeopathy works on the principle of 'like cures like' and brings the body into balance. Homeopathy uses substances found in nature to give the body the push it needs to begin healing itself.

# • Ayurvedic Medicine

Ayurvedic medicine is a very ancient holistic healing system developed thousands of years ago in India. In Ayurvedic medicine, it is believed that the root causes of infertility include nervous system imbalances, physical and mental stress, disruption of natural biological rhythms, accumulated toxins in the body, poor nutrition, sluggish digestion and a weakened immune system. In Ayurvedic medicine, it is believed that a person's physical, spiritual and emotional well-being are all interconnected.

# • Traditional Chinese Medicine

When practitioners of Chinese medicine treat infertility, they work to balance the 'foundation' of the body and the qi, or life energy, that flows through the body, through herbal medicine, acupuncture, massage, dietary therapy and exercise. Emotions, sleeping and eating habits, are all looked at in determining the root cause of infertility. They may treat infertility by suggesting increasing blood flow to the reproductive organs, through acupuncture, massage or exercise.

# Vitamins and Supplements

Here are some vitamins and supplements that can often help male infertility:

• **Vitamin C:** High-quality vitamin C supplements enhance sperm development. Some recommend 2,000 to 6,000 milligrams daily to prevent sperm from clumping or sticking together.

Foods that contain lots of Vitamin C include strawberries, citrus fruits, cherries, cantaloupe, broccoli, tomatoes, sweet peppers, mangos, kiwi, pineapple, grapes, peas, potatoes, parsley and spinach. Keep a bowl of these foods washed and easily available.

• **Zinc:** is very important to sperm quality because it increases testosterone levels, sperm count and sperm motility. Men should consider taking a zinc supplement or a high-quality multivitamin that contains zinc, as a zinc deficiency has been shown to cause or reduce male infertility.

In addition to taking a supplement, foods high in zinc include oysters, organic meats, lean beef, turkey, lamb, herring, wheat germ, beans, sunflower and pumpkin seeds.

• **L-Arginine:** is an amino acid that enhances low sperm counts and poor motility. It is found in high amounts in the head of the sperm. Studies show that sperm and semen volume double with this amino acid.

Food sources of L-arginine include nuts, raisins, sesame seeds, brown rice, peanuts, almonds chocolate, meat and poultry.

• **A Multivitamin:** taken daily.

• **Vitamin E:** Studies have shown that Vitamin E increases sperm health and motility.

• **Folic acid:** Studies suggest that men with low levels of this key B vitamin have trouble producing healthy sperm.

Folic acid reportedly improves sperm motility and sperm structure. Food sources include leafy greens, orange juice and spinach.

- **Korean Ginseng:** enhances testosterone and sperm levels.

- **Selenium:** should be taken as part of a quality multi-vitamin.

- **Coenzyme Q10:** increases energy production in the sperm and can increase motility and quality of sperm.

- **Omega-3:** acts as a hormone regulator.

- **Vitamin A:** helps enhance male hormones.

- **B-complex:** This vitamin is very important to male fertility. Vitamin B6 and B12 have been reported to improve sperm counts. Vitamin B12 can increase the quantity and quality of your guy's sperm. Foods that contain B vitamins include lamb, sardines and salmon.

- **Calcium-Magnesium:** aids Vitamin B absorption.

- **Vitamin A:** increases male hormones. Eat plenty of vegetables, fruit, oily fish and dark green leafy vegetables.

- **Royal Jelly:** can help optimize hormonal balance.

- **Manganese deficiency:** is known to result in testicular degeneration. Foods with manganese include: whole grains, green vegetables, carrots, broccoli, beans, nuts, pineapples, oats, rye and eggs.

# Things Your Guy Can Do To Improve His Fertility

• **Visit The Dentist:** Make sure your husband has his teeth cleaned, thus eliminating the possibility of infections in the gums or teeth.

• **Consider His Weight:** Too much or too little body fat can disrupt production of reproductive hormones, thus reducing sperm count. Try to help your husband/partner lose weight, especially scrotal fat, which can act like a warm blanket over the scrotum and elevate sperm temperatures, which in turn, kill and immobilize sperm. Excess fat around the waist is often associated with decreased male fertility.

• **Reduce Stress:** Encourage your husband/partner to take steps to reduce stress, as stress has been shown to negatively impact male reproductive hormones and lower testosterone.

• **Drink Lots of Water:** Make sure your partner is drinking plenty of high-quality, filtered water each day.

• **Touch, Touch and Touch Some More:** Stimulation increases hormones and improves fertility. Touch each other at length before intercourse to increase hormones, both his and yours.

• **Ejaculate Often:** Sex is good for sperm, because the less time spent in storage, the higher quality it will be and less DNA damage.

• **Enjoy More Sunshine:** Encourage your guy to get outside 10 to 15 minutes a day.

• **Balance The Body's Flora:** Eating a diet rich in nuts, seeds, fruits and vegetables can help encourage healthy sperm. Limit sugar, processed foods and encourage your guy to take a probiotic to improve digestive health and reduce inflammation. Reducing the amount of gluten consumed is also important.

• **Alkalize His Body With Greens:** Lots of healthy vegetables can help restore the acid-alkaline balance in the reproductive system to the proper sperm pH. A diet high in acid-producing foods such as meat, white flour, sugar, alcohol, coffee and soft drinks is to be avoided.

• **Nourish His Endocrine System:** The endocrine system is responsible for hormone production and secretions. Low sperm count or morphology is often caused by hormonal imbalance, and an over-stressed endocrine system.

# What Your Guy Should Avoid To Protect His Fertility

• **Keep It Loose:** Have your partner wear loose fitting boxer shorts, instead of tight underwear. Avoid boxers, briefs or bikinis.

No tight clothes around the genitals please.

• **Just Say No To Lubricants:** Avoid lubricants during sex. Lotions or lubricants can interfere with sperm motility.

• **Don't Let His Sperm Get Too Hot:** Heat can deter the healthy development of sperm. Genitals should be kept cool when possible. Lap top computers can increase scrotal temperature, which hurts sperm production.

Avoid hot tubs, saunas and Jacuzzis. Wear cotton boxer shorts rather than jockey shorts to keep sperm from overheating. Avoid long drives, and never let him put his cell phone in between his legs while driving. Avoid hot baths or overly long hot showers.

If your guy has a job that requires him to sit a lot each day, this could be causing high testicle heat. Encourage him to get up and walk every few hours.

Avoid heated car seats, electric blankets and heating pads that increase testicular temperatures—always remember sperm works better when it is cool!

If there is a chance that your partner is experiencing too much heat in his genital area, you may want to try artificially cooling his testicles with ice, a cold bath or shower. Always remember: Sperm counts are higher in the cold weather and in the morning.

• **Stop All Cigarette Smoking:** Smoking reduces sperm count and motility. It also increases the risk of genetic defects in an embryo. All smoking should be stopped.

• **No Marijuana:** Chemicals from marijuana have been reported to build up in the testicles and can cause impotence and a lower sperm count.

• **Take A Look At Prescription Drugs:** If your husband is on medication, you may want to evaluate if it is safe for him to take a break while you are trying to conceive. Some prescription drugs can negatively effect sperm count. This is a matter to be decided with a doctor's approval and notification, as some medications are absolutely necessary for various mental and physical health conditions.

• **Reduce Bicycling Activity:** Bicycling can raise scrotal temperature and critical arteries and nerves can be damaged by repeatedly banging the groin against the seat.

• **No Oral Sex:** Saliva can kill sperm. Avoid oral sex at this time.

• **No Extreme Exercise:** Extreme exercise can lower the sperm count.

• **Cut Down Or Reduce Alcohol:** Alcohol interferes with the secretion of testosterone and lowers sperm count. Alcohol can also depletes vitamins and minerals in the body and an overworked liver can cause a rise in estrogen.

• **Stay Away From Water Bottles That Contain Bisphenol A (BPA):** Be aware of Bisphenol A (known as BPA) a hormone-disrupting chemical that is a common ingredient in water bottles, canned goods, and other products. Researchers have found that men with higher urine levels of BPA have decreased sperm concentration, decreased total sperm count, decreased sperm vitality and decreased sperm motility. BPA can also be found on cash register receipts and metal cans.

• **Avoid Soaps and Deodorants That Contain Phthalates:** Phthalates are another group of chemicals that have been shown to wreak havoc with reproductive health.

They are commonly found in vinyl flooring, detergents, soap, shampoo, deodorants, fragrances, hair spray, plastic bags, vinyl shower curtains, scented soaps, cleaners, garden hoses, and sex toys.

• **Be Aware of Chemicals In His Environment:** Other chemicals that are linked to decreased fertility include: Methoxychlor and Vinclozin, an insectide and fungicide, non-fermented soy products that contain hormone-like substances, and fluoride.

Avoid plastic containers for food storage, plastic bottles, wraps and utensils.

Be aware of office paper products whitened with chlorine. Use only non-bleached coffee filters, paper, napkins and toilet tissue to reduce dioxin exposure.

• **No Chlorine Products:** Avoid chlorinated tap water, chlorine bleach and other chlorinated products.

• **No Deodorants:** Avoid synthetic deodorants and use only organic products whenever possible.

• **Reduce Cell Phone Usage and Contact:** Cell phones can negatively impact the brain's pituitary output. Ask your guy to cut down on using his phone, and tell him not to carry it in his pocket. Try to encourage him to keep wireless items that transmit EMFs away from his body.

• **Reduce WIFI Usage:** Wifi signals contain EMFs that have been found to lower sperm count.

• **No anabolic steroids**

• **Some studies suggest anti-ulcer drugs decrease sperm count**

• **Avoid Cottonseed toxins hidden in food**

• **Avoid pesticides**

• **Avoid growth hormones**

• **Reduce or Eliminate If Possible Caffeine:** Excessive amounts of caffine can impact sperm counts. Caffeine, found in tea, coffee, chocolate, cola, energy drinks, some medications, and stimulants to keep people awake, should be reduced or eliminated.

• **Reduce Contact With Lawn Care Products:** Stop using bug sprays, lawn sprays or pesticides to treat lawn and garden.

• **No More Microwaves:** Do not microwave food in plastic.

• **No Polyester:** Stop wearing polyester clothes.

# Fertility-Enhancing Foods for Men

Here are the foods your guy should eat to maximize his fertility.

• **Lots of Green Vegetables:** Green vegetables are needed to make your guy's body more alkaline. Juicing a glass of green juice each day is one way to ensure your husband has the greens he needs.

• **Spinach** is high in potassium, which improves sperm concentration.

• **Cauliflower** provides choline, that has been shown to improve sperm quality.

• **Add extra tomatoes to his salad**, as some studies have shown that the lycopene in tomatoes increase sperm count.

• **Red peppers, kiwi, lemons and strawberries** are all high in Vitamin C which has been shown to improve sperm count and motility.

• **Sardines** are rich in Omega 3's and a good source of Coenzyme Q10.

• **Avocado** has L-carnitine which promotes healthy sperm, can boost sperm motility and is packed with Vitamin E, Vitamin B6 and folic acid.

• **Pumpkin seeds** are high in zinc, loaded with omega-3 and should be a daily part of his diet.

• **Broccoli** is high in selenium

• **Wheat germ and almonds** are high in Vitamin E

• **Whole grains like oatmeal and brown rice**

• **Extra-virgin olive oil**

• **Oysters** contain a high level of zinc, which helps increase production of sperm and testosterone.

- **Brazil nuts** are rich in selenium, a mineral that boosts sperm production and mobility.

- **Walnuts** contains arginine, which increases semen volume and Omega-3s that improve blood flow to the penis.

- **Molasses**

- **Apricots**

- **Watermelon**

- **Sesame seeds**

- **Maca**

- **Spirulina**

- **Foods High In Antioxidants:** Sperm is damaged by free radicals and antioxidants can prevent cell damage. High antioxidant foods include: blueberries, blackberries, kale, garlic, Brussels sprouts, plums, red peppers, broccoli and red peppers.

- **Asparagus:** contain high amounts of Vitamin C, which prevents sperm from oxidizing and protects the cells of testes.

- **Bananas:** contain bromelain, that help increase stamina and boosts the body's ability to make sperm.

- **Wild fish**

- **Dark chocolate** contains L-Arginine, an amino acid related to the arginine in walnuts.

- **Garlic** contains allicin which increases blood flow to the genitals.

- **Pomegranate** contains an intense cocktail of antioxidants that can lower a chemical in the blood called malondialidehyde that destroys sperm.

• **Organic Free Range Meat:** Some nutritionists recommend eating organically-raised, free range meats, instead of conventional meat that contains hormones and antibiotics. Eat grass fed and organic cattle.

Conventionally raised cattle can sometimes contain high levels of hormones and antibiotics which can contribute to estrogen dominate conditions.

• **Free Range Organic Chicken:** Conventionally raised chicken is sometimes full of antibiotics and hormones which can negatively impact hormonal health.

• **Kiwi** fruit is high in zinc, which helps protect sperm from chromosomal and bacterial damage.

## Foods To Avoid or Eliminate

• Your partner should eliminate, or at least cut down, on alcohol, beer and wine while you are trying to get pregnant. Alcohol can lower sperm count, weaken sperm, and impede the secretion of testosterone. Studies have shown that alcohol can decrease sperm count for as much as three months after a big drinking fest.

• Encourage your partner to avoid sugar. Eating lots of sugar often results in hormone imbalances and robs the body of key nutrients.

• Cut down or avoid whenever possible white flour or gluten. If someone is sensitive to gluten, it can cause malabsorption of important nutrients, such as zinc, and increase inflammation throughout the body.

• Reduce or avoid foods with hydrogenated oil as much as possible.

• Reduce or avoid caffeine, which can reduce sperm count and motility. Caffeine is also detrimental to adrenal function, a gland key in productive hormones. The constant stress of caffeine can cause the body to focus on dealing with stress hormones, instead of reproductive hormones.

• Reduce or avoid animal products with a high fat content that contain hormones.

• No fried foods or hot sauce

• Avoid fried, charcoal-broiled or barbecued forms of cooking.

• Avoid soy. Soy is high in phyto estrogens, which can upset the hormonal balance in man. The estrogen-like compounds in soy can dramatically lower sperm counts. Texturized soy protein is in many meat substances used in fast food chains, and is also found in cereal, snack crackers and protein shakes.

• Avoid soda

• Stop drinking milk for now, since many dairy cows are fed estrogens to produce more milk. If you must drink milk, try to drink milk that is organic and not from estrogen-fed cows. Dairy that is not organic may contain hormones and antibiotics which can contribute to increased estrogen levels in the body. Keep dairy to a minimum.

• Avoid processed grains, GMO corn and corn products, and corn chips.

## Conditions That Might Impact Male Fertility

• Be sure your husband is aware of any food allergies he may have.

• Some cases of male infertility are linked to viruses. It would be helpful for your partner to do a parasite cleanse. Investigate whether your guy has an infection, which could be lowering his sperm count.

• Micro-organisms and bacteria may be the cause of fertility problems. Approximately 15% of cases of male factor infertility are reportedly caused by bacteria, parasites or viruses.

• Chlamydia

• Elevated prolactin levels

• Triglycerides: a sign of metabolic syndrome and insulin resistance

## One More Thing:

• There is some research that suggests that sperm levels are highest in the morning, and this could be something to speak to your doctor about when scheduling IVFs and IUI's.

## Chapter 1: The Ultimate Fertility Success Program: Getting Your Body Ready

Are you ready to be pregnant? Have you been told that you cannot get pregnant for unexplainable reasons? Have you been trying for a baby for a long time and you are weary, tired and very, very sad?

Infertility is one of the most difficult journeys a woman can take.

But, starting today, know this: Infertility is not a final statement on your ability to have the family you dream of—infertility is a medical condition that, with the right treatments, is often temporary and can be cured.

So starting today, see your infertility as a temporary condition that is a signal that your body is off-track and needs something to heal it.

Infertility clinics often give patents a diagnosis of "unexplained infertility", but infertility is never a result of unexplainable, mysterious problems. Infertility is always a result of specific problems or deficits in the body—problems that are sometimes hard to detect in the way that Western medicine diagnoses ailments.

When your body does not conceive easily and naturally, there is disease, dysfunction and malfunction occurring on some level, even if it is a level so very subtle that it cannot be detected on standardized tests.

Some of the fertility problems your body may be experiencing may be hard to find because there are not machines or diagnostic tools yet available to detect slight shifts, blocks, traumas in the body that can prevent or delay pregnancy.

So just because a doctor says you can never get pregnant does not mean your body, if helped, cannot heal from infertility—but here's the catch—you have to do the right things to get back your infertility.

By turning your body from acidic to alkaline, from a diseased toxic state to one that is cleansed, from a body full of inflammation to one that is healthy.

Sometimes, our body can get onto a disease track, and it then must be pushed and healed back over to a track of health.

In this chapter, we'll discuss a comprehensive body makeover program that will change the track you are on and help you become more healthy, vibrant and fertile—as you deserve to be!

You can go to an infertility clinic and take advantage of all the latest and best treatments and medications available, which I recommend, and at the same time embark on a course of holistic, alternative healing to maximize your chances of getting pregnant and having the babies you dream of.

The first step to overcoming infertility is to change the track your body is on from:

• A state of disease and dysfunction to one of health

• An acidic state to an alkaline state

• A state of clogged toxins in the body, to one of a cleansed body with all your organs cleansed and able to function at their highest level possible.

What can set the body down a wrong course? Unhealthy foods, low-quality drinking water, chemicals or toxins in our environment and in products we use, stress, traumas and painful life experiences that tire and weaken our organs.

Sometimes we live, eat, think and experience life in a way that can deplete our reproductive organs in ways that we are completely unaware of.

Picture yourself driving down the highway in the wrong lane. Imagine switching to another lane in order to get to your desired destination.

That is your goal right now--to get your body off the wrong road of toxic build-up to a cleansed road, from a road of tired organs to cleaned out revived organs.

Your job is to change the state of your body, by digging deep to uncover the root causes of your infertility.

Here are 10 things you can do immediately to get your body back on a healthy ready-to-conceive track:

1. Buy a juicer or a fruit/vegetable drink mixer. Learn as much as you can about making healthy vegetable and fruit drinks. Make this a daily part of your routine, whether it is simply juicing a bag of spinach or making a spinach/blueberry/flaxseed drink.

2. Find a reputable, licensed acupuncturist in your area and start going once, twice or even three times a week.

3. Visit a local health or nature food store and purchase a liver cleanse. You may want to do this more than once. This is to be done before you are in the midst of an IUI or IVF cycle.

4. Visit a supermarket and stock up on garlic, spinach, pumpkin seeds, sunflower seeds, kale, yams, and pineapple.

5. Schedule 20 minutes in your day to sit outside in the sunshine. Pick a place that feels comfortable—even if it is just putting a chair out in your front yard, a driveway or at a local park.

6. Find an excellent, highly reputable chiropractor in your area who

is somewhat familiar with issues of infertility who can adjust your spine.

7. Start eating as much spinach and garlic as you can.

8. Get more sleep. Make sure your room is completely dark and get to bed earlier.

9. Stop drinking coffee and eating sugar.

10. Stop all trans fats that are in your diet. Cut down on white flour products too.

As always check with a physician before pursuing any course of treatment.

## To begin:

**• Start by having a complete physical:** Go to your primary care physician and request a complete work-up.

You need to find out if you have:

• Gallstones

• Blood problems or disorders, such as anemia

• Ask for a complete work-up of your thyroid, liver and kidneys. This includes a thyroid stimulating hormone test and a comprehensive metabolic panel.

• Get tested for allergies, as you could be eating a food that weakens your body, such as gluten.

• Have your white blood cell count checked. This might help in determining if there is an undetected infection in your body.

The aim of the physical is to find out if there is an area in your body that has been overlooked, because one weak area can throw off the rest of the body.

**• Visit Your Dentist:** Get a complete dental check-up to be sure there are no lingering or untreated infections in your mouth.

# Cleansing and Detoxifying Your Body

## 12 Cleanses To Help Restore Your Fertility

The next step in changing the state, or condition, of your body is cleansing and detoxifying. The importance of detoxifying your body should never be underestimated. In this chapter, we'll look at 12 cleanses that can help restore and maximize your fertility potential.

Please note: cleanses should be done before you start infertility medications or treatments, because you do not want them to interfere with medications or a pregnancy, if there is even a slight chance you could be pregnant. Cleansing can be compared to overturning and fertilizing the soil before planting the seed.

If you are just starting infertility treatments, you may want to choose just one or two cleanses, so as not to delay treatment.

If you've been trying to get pregnant for a long time with no success, you might want to consider doing various cleanses to strengthen your body.

Here are some cleanses to consider:

## • A Liver Cleanse

Never never NEVER underestimate the importance of having your liver cleaned and detoxified.

The liver is a highly influential organ that plays a key role in fertility and is one of the most important organs in your body. The liver governs approximately 500 metabolic processes and many studies have shown that the oestrogen receptors in the liver are critical for maintaining fertility.

I cannot say enough about the importance of having a clean, de-toxified liver in the quest to get pregnant.

An ineffective liver allows toxins to seep into the ovaries and endocrine system.

If your liver is congested, it cannot adequately remove toxins and fats from the body.

Instead, they will continue to recirculate through your system—causing hormonal disturbances and imbalances. It also means your ovaries will be flooded with toxic substances that your liver was suppose to clean—and your ovaries are the source of your eggs. These impurities will result in poor egg quality—all because your liver was too congested to do its job. So if you want to improve the quality of your eggs, make sure your liver is as clean and detoxified as possible.

Once the liver is cleansed, the entire endocrine and reproductive system becomes free of toxins and impurities, so they can begin functioning at a higher capacity.

What causes a sluggish, tired liver? Stress, poor diet, medication, toxins in the environment, low-quality food, coffee, sugar, white flour products and low quality drinking water, are among a few of the culprits. The older we get, the more our liver needs to be cleaned out because of the junk that we have taken into our body over the years.

A liver cleanse will help kick your body into high gear, increasing energy and vitality to all your organs.

Liver cleanses can be found online and at most health and natural food stores. You may want to do a 30-day cleanse more than once.

Please note: A liver cleanse should never be done while you are taking infertility medications, as it could interfere with the effectiveness of the medication. It is something to do BEFORE you begin any infertility treatments or medication, and is never to be done if you could be pregnant.

In addition to a liver cleanse, here are some other ways to detoxify, cleanse and strengthen your liver:

• Milk thistle is a wonderful herb for cleansing the liver. Read the directions on the bottle carefully as to amounts taken.

• Lemon is a great liver cleanser. About 20 minutes before breakfast in the morning, squeeze the juice from one or two fresh lemons into some warm water and drink.

• Beets are excellent liver cleansers. You can eat them cooked or juice them. To juice beets, peel and cut into small wedges that can easily fit in your juicer. Juice the beets with some apple, spinach or kale.

• Chlorophyll is a highly esteemed liver cleanser.

• Artichokes are powerful liver protectors because they contain a flavonoid called silymarin, which is an antioxidant that protects the liver from toxicity.

• Foods that are good for your liver include: spirulina, garlic, carrots, romaine lettuce, apples, grapefruit, chicory, mustard greens, dandelion greens, avocados, walnuts, turmeric and parsley.

• Cabbage can also be juiced and is effective in cleaning the liver.

• Amino acids, derived from healthy sources of protein, are key to the liver working at maximum capacity. Foods that contain these amino acids include: nuts, such as pumpkin seeds, squash seeds and almonds; lean meats, eggs, and beans, such as lentils and garbanzo.

• In Chinese medicine, infertility is often linked to Liver chi stagnation, a result of stress, overwork, and the effects of coffee and alcohol. Irritability, headaches and frustration are just some of the physical and emotional symptoms of liver chi stagnation. Acupuncturists and herbalists can work on unblocking energy stagnation in the liver.

• According to Chinese medicine, emotional and lifestyle cures for liver stagnation include being assertive, making clear decisions and enjoying lots of fun, laughter and relaxation. Holding on to anger, feeling stuck and depression impair the liver by stagnating the energy. Letting go, moving on, and exercising control over one's life, can help in healing the liver.

## • Heavy Metal Cleanse

Every day, we come into contact with heavy metals that can disrupt our fertility. As much as possible, you'll want to start paying attention to the metals you may be unintentionally bringing into your body through the products you use and your lifestyles choices. Cosmetics, drinking soda straight from a can, deodorants that contain aluminum, solvents in dry cleaning, exposure to radiation, all contain metals that can find their way into our body, causing metabolic disruptions in organs, such as our heart, brain, kidneys and liver.

Because heavy metals are so common in our world, most of us have them in our systems. There are a variety of heavy metal cleanses available online and in health food stores. You may want to do this cleanse more than once. This is, however, a cleanse to be done before you start infertility treatments and medications.

Along with a heavy metal cleanse, here are some additional ways to cleanse your body of heavy metals:

• Garlic is known to help reduce metal levels in the body. It contains the antioxidant allicin. You can eat garlic raw, include it in your cooking or juice it. To juice, simply peel the garlic, juice, and drink combined with lemon juice and water. Have a big glass of water nearby to help reduce stomach discomfort.

• Milk thistle is an herb that can also help remove heavy metals from the liver.

• Cilantro is a powerful herb that is known for binding heavy metals and whisking them out of the body.

• Alpha Lipoic Acid and Gluthatione are powerful supplements for helping cells remove heavy metals from the body.

• Chlorella is a fresh water algae loaded with chlorophyll. Buy it in powder form and mix with water for fast absorption. It can also be taken in capsule or tablet form.

• A steam bath can help remove metals.

• Burdock is a potent blood purifier and can remove heavy metals from the body. It also helps purify the liver.

• Onions contain the antioxidant quercetin, which helps remove heavy metals from the body. Add to your salads daily or juice them.

## • A Yeast Cleanse

Yeast, also known as candida, can impact your fertility by causing your internal vagina's flora to become unbalanced, making it difficult for sperm to reach the uterus.

Candida is a common yeast that lives in our gut, and an overgrowth of it can lead to leaky gut syndrome, which wreaks havoc with many of the body's systems, including the endocrine system, that plays a huge role in reproduction and fertility

Yeast can also impact estrogen levels in the body, causing thyroid problems and hormonal imbalances. Yeast problems can come from frequent or long-term use of antibiotics, birth control pills, or eating foods with a lot of sugar. Getting rid of yeast is an important step in rebalancing your body so it can heal itself.

Some ways to rid your body of yeast:

• Do a yeast or candida cleanse, that can be bought online, at health food store or nature food store.

• Acidophillus can help control candida.

• Flaxseed is known to help control yeast.

• Garlic is an enemy of yeast. Take garlic capsules, juice garlic and eat lots of raw garlic.

• Avoid sugar and white flour foods. These can include sugary juices, desserts, breads, crackers, pre-packaged meals, soda. Be alert to foods with hidden sugar, such as salad dressings or ketchup. Avoid alcohol, chocolate, cakes and carbonated beverages.

• Eat plain yogurt.

• Consider taking probiotics in a supplement form.

• Enzyme supplements are available that are made specifically to fight yeast.

• Replace your regular salt with Celtic salt or kosher salt.

# • Adrenal Cleanse

Adrenal fatigue, also known as adrenal burn-out, impacts many women suffering with infertility. If you are having trouble getting pregnant, this could be one of the not-so-obvious and sometimes difficult to diagnose reasons behind your infertility.

The adrenals are a very important to your fertility because they are part of the endocrine system, which is responsible for producing and balancing more than 50 hormones in your body. When the adrenals are weak or not working at full capacity, the body's entire endocrine system and hormones can become imbalanced.

Adrenal burn-out occurs when the adrenals are stressed and pushed to the point where they begin producing excessive amounts of cortisol and adrenaline, which results in progesterone in the body producing too many stress hormones.

The adrenals become too sluggish, and then the other endocrine glands are not signaled to release their hormones, which results in the entire communication system in the endocrine glands breaking down.

Emotional trauma, living in a constant state of fight or flight, chemical toxins, lack of sleep, anxiety, stress, depression, poor diet, infections, and some prescription drugs, can all cause adrenal burn-out.

If the adrenals are exhausted, you may not produce enough progesterone, which is the pro-gestational hormone needed to get pregnant and carry a pregnancy to term.

Here are some ways to help strengthen your adrenals:

• Take a Vitamin C supplement. The adrenal gland uses vitamin C at a higher rate than other cells in the body.

• Don't let your blood sugar levels get too low. Eat regular meals and never skip breakfast. Keep your blood sugar levels normal by eating healthy foods throughout the day.

• Stop drinking coffee or drink no more than one cup of coffee a day. Caffeine depletes the body of B vitamins, which the adrenals need. Stop trying to energize and push your body by drinking another cup of coffee. Instead, eat fruits and vegetables that will provide your body with healthy forms of energy.

• Drink lots of high-quality water.

• Consider taking a Vitamin B complex, Vitamin E and an adrenal gland supplement.

• A high-quality liquid trace mineral supplement can help support the adrenal glands. Note: Although you may want to drastically reduce your intake of this supplement once you are pregnant, or consult with a doctor on the levels of minerals that are safe and healthy to take during pregnancy.

• Make lifestyle changes that reduce stress in your life. Do you need to change jobs? Relocate? Take a hard and honest look at the way you live your daily life. Start including more activities in your life that eliminate stress and reduce a fight-or-flight way of living. These include: deep breathing, massage, daily walks by a lake, ocean or in a beautiful park.

Consider more time for prayer, journal writing, and positive visualization.

• Foods that help adrenals include spinach, garlic, onions, green leafy vegetables and brown rice.

• Almonds and cashews, which are high in magnesium, are very healthy for the adrenal system.

• Eat more seeds, such as sunflower and pumpkin seeds.

• Avoid white flour products, soda, sugary fruit juices or anything that makes blood sugar levels rise rapidly.

• Alternative health therapies, such as applied kinesiology, myofascial release, and craniosacral therapy can restore a weakened adrenal system.

• Getting more sleep and better sleep can help restore the adrenal glands. So, go to bed earlier, preferably aim for a 9 to 10 o'clock bedtime, and try to stop all technology and electronic stimulation about an hour before bed for a better quality sleep.

• Sea salt, celtic salt or regular salt in moderate amounts can help the adrenal system provided that you don't suffer from high-blood pressure.

• Healthy fats like olive oil, coconut oil, ground flax seed or flax seed oil are excellent for burnt-out and exhausted adrenals.

• Adrenal exhaustion can sometimes be caused by hidden food allergies. Find out if you are allergic to wheat, corn or dairy products.

## • A Colon Cleanse

Cleansing your colon can significantly improve your overall health and fertility. A colon that is diseased, inflamed or full of yeast, mold, fungus or parasites can cause a general malaise in the body and lower the body's pH balance, making it more acidic – and acid creates a hostile environment for reproductive health.

A colon that is weighed down by years of buildup can also press on the uterus and surrounding reproductive organs.

Those who have undergone colon cleanses will attest to the dramatic improvements in how they feel afterwards. By ridding your body of decaying matter, you could very well be turning back the hands of time. Colon cleansing, sometimes called colon hydrotherapy, can rid the body of chemicals and toxins that affect the egg and sperm.

Colonic irrigation and herbal cleansings help remove toxins, parasites and mucus that have built up in the colon. By flushing out impacted waste, passing stool is easier and transit times are improved. Removing impurities goes a long way in helping the body absorb nutrients, and enhancing energy levels.

Some doctors believe that poor bowel management is at the root of many health problems, and many diseases are a result of toxins built-up in the intestinal tract that are not eliminated. A digestive tract that has a build-up of unhealthy, slow moving foods that stick to the intestinal walls result in an overburdened colon full of decaying fecal matter and foods are acid-forming.

Yeasts, molds, fungus, bacteria, parasites and fecal materal can then enter the blood stream, causing what is known as leaky bowel syndrome.

This results in a reduction of nutrients the body is able to absorb, and in turn impacts fertility.

Have your colon cleansed, at a licensed, reputable establishment with a long-time track record.

This can be an uncomfortable process, but in cleaning out your colon, you will be bringing new youth to your body.

You can also clean your colon with colon cleansing products available online, or at a natural foods store or supermarket.

Note: once there is even a chance that you are pregnant, stop all colon cleanses. This is something to be done only BEFORE there is any chance you are pregnant. If there is any possibility that you are pregnant, do not continue with any type of colon cleanse.

Here are some other ways to cleanse and detoxify your colon:

• Foods that help keep the colon clean include apples, blackberries, blueberries, raspberries, figs, dates, avocados, spinach, Swiss chard, oatmeal, flax, and chickpeas.

• Foods to avoid include sugar, white flour, and hormone/antibiotic-filled meats that assault the body.

• Fennel and garlic are known to kill bacteria and parasites in the colon, thus improving colon function.

• Cayenne pepper and garlic are also known colon cleansers.

• Flaxseeds and psyllium husk seeds help clean the colon.

• Herbs like Slippery Elm and Cascara Sagrada also are used in many colon detoxification cleanses.

• Eat large amounts of fiber.

• Ginger and garlic can help with healthy bowel movements, along with some olive oil in the morning. Leafy greens and healthy fibers can also aid in elimination.

• Apples and carrots, which contain a large amount of water, go far in cleansing the colon.

• Consider juicing apples, carrots, spinach, and other green vegetables as a way to help cleanse the colon.

• Be aware of your bowel movements. Make sure you are having at least one healthy bowel movement a day. Don't hold in a bowel movement if you feel it coming.

• Drink lemon, honey or maple syrup and cayenne pepper several times a day. Drink with or without food for several days as a way to cleanse the colon.

• Reduce the amount of processed foods, fast foods, pizza and foods with additives that you eat.

• While detoxifying your colon, start taking probiotics as a way to replenish your intestinal flora.

• Eat a diet with a lot of high fiber vegetables, such as dark leafy greens,

• Drink a lot of high-quality water each day. Inadequate hydration can lead to a build-up of toxins in the colon.

• Juice or make a drink with vegetables daily.

• Include essential fatty acids in your diet, such as ground flax seed, evening primrose oil, cod liver oil and coconut oil.

• Eat foods rich in healthy fats, such as avocados, olive oil and nuts.

• Include more olive oil in your diet, because it reduces bile acid and increase enzymes that regulate cell turn over in the lining of the intestines.

• In Chinese medicine, the colon is one of the two organs in the metal element, and has the function of eliminating what is unnecessary or toxic in our bodies. On the emotional level, the colon enables us to let go of the garbage directed at our bodies and spirit. To heal the colon, it is important to 'let go' of negative experiences that may have tainted our self-worth.

For issues that are unresolved, write them on paper and burn them, thus releasing their content. Breath slowly and deeply each day. As you breath, feel the negativity, impurity and pain leave your body, and breath in energized, purified air. If you are chronically constipated, it may be that you are having a hard time letting go of something in your life, such as a past hurt, rejection or trauma. Allow yourself to accept and be open to new experiences in your life. As much as you can, make room for new, transforming experiences in your life.

## • Kidney Cleanse

According to Chinese herbal medicine, one of the most common causes of infertility is a problem with or a deficiency in the kidney. In fact, in Chinese medicine, a kidney deficiency is the most common diagnosis in infertility.

In Chinese medicine, the kidney is considered the main root of our Qi (chi) which regulates reproduction and is considered the seat of procreation, the vitality center of the body. A weak Qi, or kidney function, affects the quality and development of eggs, and impacts the ovaries and uterus.

A kidney deficiency is often a result of poor diet and stress.

Here are various ways to cleanse and strengthen the kidney:

• Make sure you are working on cleansing and detoxifying the liver, because a healthy, clean liver results in a healthy, strong kidney.

• Find an acupuncturist who is experienced in working with kidney deficiency and its impact on fertility.

• Stop all coffee or limit coffee intake to no more than a cup a day.

• Avoid carbonated beverages, artificial sweeteners and excessive amounts of dairy products.

• Limit red meat.

• Reduce sugar and sodium in your diet. Stop potato chips, crackers, cheese spreads, deli meats and instant potato mixes.

• Kidney problems are often the result of stress, chronic anger and shame, so it is important to release and free yourself from these feelings. Journal writing, prayer, forgiveness of yourself and others, are all steps that can begin the healing process.

• Dandelion tea is known to help flush toxins from the kidney.

• Cod liver oil contains high levels of Vitamin D that strengthen the kidneys.

• Foods that regenerate the kidney include chestnuts, strawberries, walnuts, raspberries; black, kidney and mung beans, fennel, onions, beetroot, garlic, ginger, cloves, red bell peppers, cabbage, cauliflower, dandelion, blueberries, red grapes, and wild salmon.

• Add lots of flaxseed, pumpkin, and sunflower seeds to your diet.

• Walnuts and chestnuts enhance the kidney's function.

• Spirulina, kelp, chlorella, and wheatgrass are good for the kidney.

• Eat lots of asparagus and other deep green leafy vegetables.

• The herb Nettle is known to strengthen the kidney.

• Drink lots of water.

• Limit alcohol intake. Do not overtax your kidney with too much alcohol.

- Juice cabbage, parsley, cucumbers and ginger.

- Eat more apples, cranberries, olive oil, and onions.

- Stay away from high-sodium foods.

- Milk thistle is a great nutrient for the kidney.

- Staying hydrated is very important to flushing out toxins in the kidney.

- Eat large amounts of watermelon for a few days.

- A Chinese herbalist can provide herbal formulas to clean the kidney.

- Burdock tea helps removes waste from the kidneys.

- Dandelion tea is known to help cleanse the kidneys.

- Ginger root and turmeric tea is good for the kidneys and can be made by boiling some turmeric powder with peeled ginger root.

- Grapes and cranberries. Grapes help flush uric acid and other waste products from the kidney. Cranberries contain quinine, which the liver converts to hippuric acid, which in turns helps remove urea and uric acid from the kidneys.

- Apples are often used as a home remedy for kidney stones.

- Garlic is a natural diuretic that helps flush out kidneys.

- Cucumbers are a natural diuretic that can dissolve kidney and bladder stones.

- Onions can help pass kidney stones.

- Kidney beans and peas contain arginine, an amino acid that helps cleanse the kidney of ammonia.

• Make sure you are getting enough Vitamin C, Vitamin E, calcium and B-6.

• Keep your blood pressure, blood glucose level, and cholesterol levels in healthy ranges, so your kidneys are not overtaxed.

• According to natural healers, the emotion that seems to impact the kidney the most is fear. Some believe that chronic fear and anxiety in childhood impacts the health of the kidneys later in life. To release fear, begin to embrace your life with courage. Welcome life! Do not push it away or hid from it.

In Chinese medicine, the ability to use our will power to express our unique creativity is also dependent on good kidney energy. With a strong kidney qi, we will have the resolve to overcome fear and pursue goals. A weak kidney results in a shaky sense of purpose and one who is easily distracted. Feeling stuck and not letting go is also sometimes the emotional root of kidney disease. The kidneys can store deep sadness, which can in turn result in illness. It is important to work on letting go of anger, fear, and traumatic, painful memories. Bring balance into your life in whenever way you can. Enjoy natural beauty and lots of rest. Spend more time enjoying natural bodies of water, such as lakes, oceans, and rivers. Keep a bowl of water with flowers nearby.

• Get a foot massage. Ask the massage therapist to stimulate and massage the kidney point on the foot that will revitalize the kidney qi.

## • Parasite Cleanse

Another facet of cleansing is eliminating parasites in your body. Parasites can impact hormone levels and some nutritionists feel that parasites can also weaken a man's sperm quality.

Symptoms of parasites include brain fog or mental fuzziness, toe fungus or athletes foot, constant illness, rectal itching, especially at night, endometriosis, anxiety and depression.

Sleep problems, immune disorders, teeth grinding, eczema, hives, and chronic fatigue can also be the result of parasites.

Common tests that can discover whether or not you have parasites include a comprehensive digestive stool analysis, candida testing and a gastric acid self-test.
Doctors can also test for parasites through x-rays.

To avoid getting parasites, do not eat raw fish or sushi and be sure to cook all fish very well. Avoid undercooked meat. Wash all fruits and vegetables thoroughly. Be very careful when eating at salad bars. Do not let animals lick you in the face or mouth. Be aware of foods you eat when you visit other countries.

Health food stores and various health-related web sites have various parasite cleanses to choose from, and this is often a first and best step to rid the body of parasites. Make sure to drink lots of water while cleansing.

Along with doing a parasite cleanse, here are some tips on ridding your body of parasites:

• Pineapple is an effective agent in ridding the body of parasites. Pineapple contains the digestive enzyme bromelain that can help clear tapeworms.

• The probiotics in yogurt are also known to kill parasites.

• Avoid sugar. Parasites are known to feed off sugar—so the less that is in your system, the less they are able to flourish within your body.

• Avoid or reduce white flour products.

• Apple cider vinegar, which is high in B-vitamins, can help neutralize the body's pH balance and improve digestion.

• Probiotics can help restore gut bacteria wiped out by parasites. Do not take a probiotic, however, within an hour of taking apple cider vinegar.

• Cinnamon is a natural remedy for parasites.

• Include more garlic in your diet. Juice it, eat it, include it in your meals, whenever you can.

• Olive oil can help remove parasite waste.

• Trichomoniasis is a vaginal infection that is seen to play a role in infertility. Ask to be tested for this.

• Chlorphyl can help eliminate parasites.

• Papaya seeds are a natural method for removing parasites. Blend them with honey or coconut oil for seven days in a row, as a parasite cleanse. Make sure to drink lots of water while cleansing.

• Pumpkin seeds are effective in killing roundworms or tapeworms. Oven roast lightly. They are more effective if eaten on an empty stomach.

• Eat pomegranates alone as they are known for destroying worms in the intestinal tract.

• Cloves and turmeric can help fight parasites.

• Sweet potatoes and squash can increase resistance to parasites because of their high Vitamin A content.

• Raw onions and garlic provide sulfur containing amino acids that are anti-parasitic.

• Thyme and thyme tea can help clear the body of parasites.

• Cayenne pepper helps repel parasites.

• A colonic irrigation, also known as a colon cleaning, can also help kill parasites.

# • Uterine Cleanse

You want to do everything possible to create the best and healthiest environment for your growing baby, and that means doing what is needed to create a healthy uterine lining for implantation of your embryos.

Conditions like hormonal imbalance, low circulation, or an unhealthy diet can impact the uterus. Other factors that impact the condition of the uterus include: stagnation of blood flow to the uterus, uterine fibroids, scar tissue from a cesarean, abdominal surgery, a D&C after a miscarriage, endometriosis, or a pelvic inflammatory disease caused by a sexually transmitted disease.

Here are some ways to cleanse and strengthen your uterus:

• Goldenseal root cleanses the uterus.

• Dong Quai, an herb, increases blood flow to the uterus and builds the uterine lining. It also tones and strengthens the uterus by regulating hormonal balance, improving uterine tone and is a blood tonic that helps circulation. It also relieves congestion and pain in the reproductive system.

• Damiana, an herb, encourages circulation and blood supply to the uterus.

• Red Raspberry Leaf or Red Raspberry Root has long been used as a uterine tonic to regulate and tone uterine muscles. It can be taken as a supplement or a tea.

• Eat or juice dandelion leaves, spinach, beets, garlic and lemon.

• Nettle Leaves is a uterine cleanser.

• L-Arginine promotes synthesis of nitric oxide, which increases blood flow to the uterus and ovaries.

• Eating foods rich in zinc can help strengthen the uterus. These include pumpkin seeds, sesame seeds and spinach.

• Some health practitioners recommend propping one's legs up against a wall 15 minutes a day to encourage increased blood flow to the uterus.

• Avoid soy and peas.

• Acupuncture can help bring more blood to your uterus. Let your acupuncturist know you are working on fertility and would like to improve your circulation to your uterus.

• Eat blood nourishing foods, such as spinach and dates.

• Pomegranates and pomegranate juice can help build uterine lining.

• Chinese medicine adheres to the belief that it is important to keep the uterus and belly warm while trying to get pregnant. They suggest not drinking or eating anything too cold, wearing socks and keeping one's feet warm at night. Do not go barefoot or wear flip-flops.
However, this does not mean overheating your body with a water bottle or doing anything that could overheat a growing fetus.

• Write a letter to your womb. Let whatever wants to be said come up and be said. Express whatever you are feeling, whether it is anger, fear or lack of self-love. Do not repress any of your feelings. Allow yourself the freedom to speak your truth, whatever it is.

• Practice deep breathing into your uterus and repeat the affirmation: I receive, I receive, I receive. I receive my baby, I receive my baby, I receive my baby.

• Your uterus deserves acknowledgement, respect and unconditional love. It needs to be told it is strong enough, good enough and worthy enough to receive a baby.

• A Native American fertility tradition is to wear a long skirt with no underwear, and sit on the ground to release whatever wounds are within you into the earth. As you do this, imagine your womb is a beautiful flowering place full of energy and light. Let the earth's energy flow up to your uterus, so it can draw from the healing energy of the earth.

• Pineapple contains a proteolytic enzyme called bromelain which reduces inflammation and breaks up proteins that prevent embryo implantation. Eating pineapple core a few days before and after an IVF cycle can help implantation. But stop eating pineapple immediately after any IVF or IUI or if you think if there is any chance you might be pregnant. While pineapple helps implantation, it is definitely not recommended for pregnancy.

• Eat lots of blueberries. Research shows they contain anthocyanins that help maintain the lining of the uterus.

• Brazil nuts contain selenium, that can thicken the uterine lining and help with implantation.

• Foods with omega-3 fatty acids can improve blood flow to the uterus, such as salmon, flaxseed oil, pumpkin seeds, walnuts, and olive oil.

• See a massage therapist who is familiar with massage to help increase circulation to the uterus and unblock the reproductive system. Look for a massage therapist experienced in deep tissue massage or massage that is used to clear blocked energy in the organs.

Acupressure, myofacial release and reflexology can also offer massage that brings blood and oxygen to the reproductive organs.

• Ask your uterus these questions: have you ever felt judged? Blamed? Abused? What do you need to heal? What can I do to help you feel loved and nurtured? Write the answers that come up from within you.

• Visualize your uterus as a cozy, warm, loving and safe place for your baby. Repeat, write and sing these affirmations:
-my uterus is healthy and just right for my baby
-my uterus welcomes my baby
-my uterus is a safe and welcoming place for my baby
-my uterus is a healing, balanced, and loving home for my baby
-I love you uterus. Thank you for taking good care of my baby.
-Uterus, you are enough. You are enough to hold my baby.
-Dear uterus, I honor and respect you.

• Supplements recommended to help implantation include zinc, Vitamin C, selenium and iron.

• Important To Note: herbs used to strengthen and cleanse your uterus must be stopped once there is any chance you are pregnant or while taking infertility medications.


## • Blood Cleanse

You want to cleanse your blood of toxins and chemicals as much as possible, because chemicals and toxins in your bloodstream can impact the health of your eggs and various organs that impact fertility.

Here are some ways to cleanse and detoxify your blood:

• Chlorophyll is known to cleanse the blood of impurities.

• Juice or eat cilantro, parsley and beets. Beet juice is a strong blood purifier.

• Drink lemon and water


• Burdock Root is revered by natural practitioners as one of the most effective blood cleansers and purifiers.It strengthens the liver and increases urination to help the kidneys remove toxins from the blood.

• Yellow Dock Root enriches and purifies the blood

• Dandelion promotes bile production that breaks down fats in the body, and destroys harmful microbes found in digested food that can enter the bloodstream.

• Goji berries are a powerful antioxidant that alkalize the blood.

• Consider digestive enzymes between meals or before bed

• Red clover is a blood purifier.

• Apple cider vinegar helps cleanse the blood.

• Echinacea is known for enhancing the immune system and cleaning the blood of pathogens.

• Drink lots of pure water

• Garlic is a strong blood purifier. Juice it, eat it, crush cloves of garlic in water and drink it, or chew on raw garlic each day.

• Turmeric purifies the blood

• Teas made from Oregon Grape Root and Sarsaparilla Root rid the blood of waste products.

• Broccoli, cabbage, cauliflower and watercress are all blood purifiers. Some recommend juicing cauliflower as a great way to clean your blood.

• Parsley is a natural blood cleanser.

• Cayenne pepper improves the circulatory system by cleaning out the channels that the blood flows through.

# • A Lymph System Cleanse

The lymph is a very important, but often overlooked, system in the body that impacts fertility.

It is so important that some health practitioners believe that a clogged, sluggish, toxic lymph system accounts for many illnesses in the body.

The lymph system is a complex system of vessels and ducts that move fluid and toxins out of the body. A sluggish lymph system means the body is not disposing of waste properly. This affects fertility because the lymphatic system plays a key role in the circulation of hormones, and a stagnant lymphatic system can impact the feedback system of these hormones.

A cleansed lymph system can help revive sluggish, congested ovaries and reduce acid levels in the vagina.

Lack of exercise, a sedentary lifestyle, stress, chronic digestive imbalances, and a high-sodium diet, can make the lymphatic system sluggish and ineffective.

Symptoms of a sluggish lymph system include feeling tired and fatigued, getting sick a lot, being overweight, having fatty deposits of cellulite, acne, rashes, as well as having lots of food sensitivities and allergies.

Some believe that fibromyalgia and chronic fatigue syndrome are a result of a clogged lymph system.

Here are some ways to cleanse the lymph system:

• To help the flow of your lymph system, drink plenty of high-quality water each day. Staying well hydrated is key to a healthy lymph system.

• Eliminate, as much as you can, sugar, soda and fruit juices from your diet.

• Always remember that the lymph system has no pump, so it is up to you to help keep your lymph flowing by drinking lots of water and moving your body. Exercises such as jumping on a mini-trampoline, dancing, walking or swimming are helpful. Jumping helps the lymphatic circulation by stimulating the millions of one-way valves in the system. If you are laid up due to a surgery or illness, it is important to find ways to move the lymph system, such as a lymph massage of a self-massage.

• Do deep breathing exercises.

• Eat lots of green vegetables to purify the blood and lymph.

• Essential fatty acids are important to the lymph. Walnuts and flaxseeds give the lymph system the fatty acids it needs. Almonds, sunflower seeds, pumpkin seeds, Brazil nuts, coconut oil and flaxseed oil also provide essential fatty acid.

• Use a natural bristle brush to brush your skin in circular motions, upward from the feet to the torso, before showering.

• Avoid processed foods that have artificial preservatives, flavors, colors, stabilizers, which includes many packaged and fast foods. These can also include hot dogs, canned foods, cereals, packaged dinners and luncheon meats.

• Avoid fatty foods and white breads.

• Raw fruit is a powerful lymph cleanser.

• Cranberries and cranberry juice can also help emulsify fat in the lymph system.

• Foods that help the lymph system include beets, onions, garlic, avocados, seaweed, kelp, kombu, kale, radish and mustard greens.

• Juice one green drink a day.

• Eat lots of citrus fruits, like lemons and limes.

• Take chlorophyll to help purify your lymph system.

• Consider an apple cider vinegar cleanse that combines honey, garlic and apple cider in a blender.

• Herbs such as Echinacea, Goldenseal and Astragalus can lessen congestion and swelling in the lymphatic system.

• One of the ways to cleanse your lymph system is a lymphatic massage, sometimes called manual lymphatic drainage.

Lymph massage is a very gentle form of deep tissue massage that moves the lymph under your skin, freeing trapped toxins and improves lymph flow in the body. It combines a gentle pressure with soft pumping movements in the direction of the lymph nodes in the body. You can find this type of practitioner by searching 'lymphatic drainage massage with your city/town/' or by searching holistic practitioners in your area, who might be able to direct you to someone who does this type of massage.

• Massaging under your arms can be helpful in relieving congestion. Place your fingertips under your armpit. Then gently push inward, towards the center of your body. Repeat this circular motion.

• Acupuncture is very helpful to the lymph system.

• Drink a cup of red clover tea each day.

• Laugh from your belly, which helps pump your lymphatic system.

• Avoid white flour products, white rice, bread and pasta, as much as possible.

• Eating foods high in potassium can improve your lymph system. These include bananas, raisins, dates, spinach and orange juice.

• Sip hot water throughout the day.

• Beets are healthy for the lymph system.

• Cayenne pepper can boost a sluggish lymph system and reduce mucous congestion.

• Stop using underarm deodorants that contain aluminium and clog the natural excretion of toxins from the lymph system.

• Stop wearing tight bras.

• Letting yourself feel your congested emotions encourages natural detoxification of the lymph system. Allow yourself to feel. Let yourself express your grief through crying, moving anger out of your body, talking, writing or whatever way your body chooses. Honor and express your emotions.

# • Thyroid Cleanse

Your thyroid is a key organ that impacts your fertility.

To keep your thyroid healthy:

• As much as possible, eliminate gluten from your diet.

• Alkalize your body as much as possible, through green vegetables, green drinks and green smoothies.

• Drink warm lemon water throughout the day to loosen toxins in the digestive system.

• Foods that can help the thyroid include: Spirulina, Brazil nuts, sunflower seeds, black walnuts.

• Iodized table salt

• Chlorophyl and coconut oil are known to strengthen the thyroid.

• Avoid all soy products

• Herbs to consider include Irish moss and Kelp.

**Excerpt from Dancing Your Way to Fertility, available on Amazon.com.**

# Balancing Your Hormones and Improving the Quality of Your Eggs

## • Balancing Your Hormones

If our hormones are not balanced, our fertility is compromised on every level. Our hormones, produced by our glands and tissues, are chemical communicators that deliver messages to our body. These messages are then released into our blood, where they travel to other tissues and send signals initiating various activities within our body and brain.

Hormones affect how we think and feel.

Our hormones are impacted by stress, fluid changes in the body, vitamin and mineral levels, infections, exposure to environmental toxins and body fat. Blood sugar imbalances, a toxic liver, folic acid deficiency, inflammation in the ovaries, breast and joints, and unhealthy gut flora can all be a result of unbalanced hormones.

Other symptoms of a hormonal imbalance can include insomnia, headaches, migraines, anxiety, foggy thinking, hot flashes, mood swings, thinning hair, bloating, rapid heartbeat, and allergies. Our hormones are impacted by stress, fluid changes in the body, vitamin and mineral levels, infection and exposure to environmental toxins and body fat.

It is important to support and strengthen the entire endocrine system. Hormones are coordinated by this system, which includes the hypothalamus, pituitary gland, adrenal gland, thyroid, parathyroid, pancreas, pineal gland, thymus and ovaries.

The foods you eat, the stress levels you experience, the chemicals in your environment, all impact the endocrine system, and in turn, your hormones.

Progesterone is a key hormone in fertility and you want to do whatever you can to make sure you have adequate progesterone levels in your body. Progesterone plays an important role in conception and maintaining a healthy pregnancy. It works to balance the effects of estrogen.

It helps maintain the lining of the uterus, which makes it possible for a fertilized egg to attach and survive.

It also makes cervical mucous accessible to the sperm, preventing immune rejection of the developing baby and normalizes blood clotting. Progesterone is produced by the corpus luteum in the ovaries and by the adrenal glands.

One of the main causes of a progesterone defiency is too much estrogen in the body. Estrogen dominance is extremely dangerous to one's fertility. It can result from eating a lot of commercially raised meat and dairy products that contain large amounts of estrogen. Chemicals called xenoestrogens are often in these food sources and they mimic the hormone estrogen and disrupt the delicate balance between estrogen and progesterone. Other excess hormones and hormone-like substances found in our environment, food and water also impact progesterone levels in the body. Pollution, stress, processed foods, soy products, and endometriosis, can cause an overload of estrogen. Allergies like asthma, hives, dry eyes, weight gain, irregular periods, and foggy thinking are symptoms of estrogen dominance.

A low thyroid, recurrent early miscarriages, sleep disturbances, and heart palpitations, can sometimes be symptoms of progesterone deficiency.

Other hormones important to fertility include estradiol, or estrogen, that are produced by the follicles and corpus luteum, also known as the remnant egg sac in the ovaries.

The luteinizing hormone, known as the LH surge, produced in the anterior pituitary gland, triggers ovulation and the development of the corpus luteum. It works in conjunction with the follicle stimulating hormone (FSH) that is also released and synthesized by the anterior pituitary gland. The FSH hormone regulates the reproductive process and signals the follicles in the ovary to begin maturing in preparation for ovulation.

Tests that can track your hormone levels include progesterone, estradiol, FSH, LH, prolactin, testosterone, sex hormone binding globulin, glucose tolerance test, thyroid panel and a blood lipid panel.

Here are some ways to balance and maintain healthy fertility hormone levels in your body:

• Reduce your exposure to xenohormones, which can be found in car exhaust, plastics, solvents, adhesives, pesticides, and emulsifiers found in soap and cosmetics and PCD's from industrial waste.

• Consider the herb Chaste Tree Berry, also known as Vitex Extract, that can balance hormones and strengthen the pituitary and ovary glands. This herb can correct hormonal communication in the body and hormonal problems at their source.

• Progesterone shots. You may want to talk to your doctor about progesterone shots if you had recurrent miscarriages or just want help maintaining your pregnancy. This is something to consider requesting if your doctor has not initiated it and if you exhibit the symptoms of a progesterone deficiency.

• Natural progesterone cream. Check with your doctor and discuss the amount to use.

• Vitamin B6 is known to help maintain optimal levels of progesterone and is key in progesterone production. Vitamin B also helps the liver break down estrogen. Food sources of Vitamin B6 can be found in walnuts, lean red meat, poultry, bananas, spinach, and potatoes.

• Turmeric, thyme and oregano are all considered helpful in raising progesterone levels.

• Vitamin C is known to considerably increase progesterone production.

• Zinc is key for producing adequate levels of progesterone in the body. That is because Zinc is a mineral that prompts the pituitary gland to release follicle stimulating hormones, which in turn promote ovulation and stimulate the ovaries to produce estrogen and progesterone. Along with a zinc supplement, natural sources of zinc include lean red meats, wheat germ, chickpeas, pumpkin and squash seeds, watermelon and dark chocolate.

• Practice stress-reduction techniques, as stress can considerably reduce progesterone levels in the body.

• Do you have low cholesterol? This can mean you are not making enough pregnenolone, which is used to make progesterone.

• Are your adrenals healthy? They house DHEA that is essential to the production of progesterone. One way to improve your adrenal health is to improve your natural circadian rhythm and get more sleep.

• Maintain a healthy digestive tract. If you have a damaged digestive tract, you won't have the raw materials within your body to absorb the nutrients in your food that helps the body produce hormones.

• You may want to consider testing for parasites, candida, or pathogens which can impact your hormonal balance.

• Maca, a root vegetable in the radish family, can balance hormones and nourish and balance the endocrine system. It protects the body from stress damage. Maca is a nutritionally dense super food that contains high amounts of minerals, vitamins, enzymes and all of the essential amino acids. Maca also stimulates and nourishes the hypothalamus and pituitary glands, which are the "master glands" of the body. It is available in powder form or capsules.

• Coconut oil stimulates the thyroid and provides omega-3's that help balance hormones. Other healthy fats essential to hormone health include flax oil, evening primrose oil and olive oil.

• Magnesium is known to break down excessive estrogens in the system and assist in balancing hormones. Kelp and cashews are rich in magnesium. Other sources of magnesium include black beans, spinach, okra, watermelon seeds, sunflower, pumpkin seeds and squash seeds.

• Garlic is an important nutrient for the endocrine system.

• Ginkgo and ginseng help regulate hormones

• Consider supplements such as Vitamin C and Vitamin B.
• Getting more sleep helps balance hormones.

• Flaxseed contains lignans and fiber, which help remove excess estrogen from the body.

• Hormone imbalances can be a result of obesity. Fat cells can create hormonal imbalances. If you think you are overweight, consider trying to lose some of the weight to help your hormonal system.

• Red Clover, an herb, protects the body from xenohormones.

• Black Cohosh, an herb, is well-known for its effect on hormone functioning.

• Do a liver cleanse. The liver plays a key role in to hormonal balance. Milk thistle, dandelion leaf and burdock root are all potent liver cleansers.

• Royal jelly is rich in amino acids and contains acetylcholine, which is needed to transmit nerve messages from cell to cell.

• Ashwagandha root supports endocrine system function and helps to regulate hormones.

• Be aware of chemicals in your diet, water, and environment that can throw your hormones out of balance.

• Drink only filtered water. Avoid water with fluoride. Fluoride is known to weaken the thyroid, one of the key organs responsible for your hormones.

• Be aware of products that may contain aluminium, including deodorants, anti-perspirants, and cosmetics.

• Be careful of meats coated with nitrate salts.

• Do not eat foods from plastic containers. Whenever possible, use glass and stainless steel.

• Avoid vegetable oil, canola oil, soybean oil, margarine, shortening and other chemically altered fats.

• Drink whole milk, not skim milk

• Licorice is a hormone balancer.

• Natural sources of iodine can help regulate hormones. These include kelp, cranberries and strawberries.

• Improve indoor air-quality with plants.

• Limit caffeine.

• Other supplements to consider for hormonal balance include calcium, Vitamin E and grapeseed extract.

• Address your hormonal imbalance on the emotional level. Are you feeling trapped? Unloved? Stuck? Angry? Are you living in a way that is true to who you are? Let your body tell you why your hormones are imbalanced.

- **Foods To Help Balance Hormones**

- Pumpkin seeds and Brazil nuts.

- Avocados and acai

- Spinach, kale, parsley, broccoli, asparagus and other leafy greens.

- Sweet peppers.

- Pears and peaches are known to help regulate hormones. They are used often in traditional Chinese medicine.

- Shiitake and reishi mushrooms, chia seeds, seaweed and spirulina.

- Avocados block estrogen absorption and promote progesterone production.

# How to Improve Your Egg Quality

Good news—you can improve the health and quality of your eggs.

In the past, we were told we were all born with a certain number of egg cells that run out as we age. We were led to believe that egg cells were the only cells in the body that did not regenerate, but instead were a finite number. We are finding out THIS IS JUST NOT TRUE. Recent research has shown that women can produce new eggs throughout their reproductive years.

You may have been told that your eggs are not healthy or that your eggs are too old.

Here's the great news: there is much you can do to enhance the health of your eggs.

It was commonly believed that the only factor that determined egg health and quality was age. Several new studies have shown that stress, hormones and environmental toxins all impact our egg health.

Your egg's health is a key cornerstone of a healthy fertility, because the health of your eggs can affect whether or not fertilization, implantation and ultimately a healthy pregnancy and birth will occur.

Here are some things you can do to improve your egg health:

• Coenzyme Q10: Coenzyme Q10 is an excellent way to improve the quality and energy within your eggs. In several studies, the supplement Coenzyme Q10 has been shown to improve egg quality. It boosts energy production in the oocytes, which are cells in the ovary. Providing additional energy in the form of Coenzyme Q10 is needed when there is decreased energy production in the ovaries due to aging. It is also a source of fuel for the mitochondria, which produces energy within the cells and with age, can begin to weaken. Along with taking a Coenzyme Q10 supplement, natural sources of CoQ10 include almonds, spinach, sardines, broccoli, strawberries, and walnuts.

• Green Tea: Green Tea contains hypoxanthine which provides follicular fluid that helps eggs mature, along with polyphenols that are powerful antioxidants that prevent chromosomal abnormalities, and repair oxidative damage within the body. However, green tea can reduce the body's absorption of folic acid, so you may want to increase your dosage of folic acid at the same time.

• Start eating foods high in antioxidants that will protect your eggs from free radical damage. Free radicals can damage both the egg cell health and the cell's DNA. Foods high in antioxidants that can combat free radicals include blueberries, cranberries, garlic, Granny apples, artichokes, spinach, kale, broccoli, plums, walnuts, and oregano.

• Include Maca in your diet, which is a root-like cruciferous vegetable and the only plant known in the world that can grow and thrive at a high altitude in harsh weather. Maca contains 31 different minerals and 60 different phytonutrients. It nourishes the endocrine system, aids the pituitary, adrenal and thyroid glands, and helps balance hormones and increases energy and stamina in the body.

Maca controls estrogen levels in the body, which is very important because if estrogen levels are too high or low, it can prevent a woman from becoming pregnant or carrying full term. Excess estrogen levels can also cause progesterone levels to become low. Make sure that when you purchase Maca, it contains the root, not just leaves and stem. Once, you are pregnant, you need to stop Maca immediately—it is to be taken only to prepare your body to become pregnant.

• L-Arginine is an amino acid that has been shown to increase ovarian response, endometrial receptivity and pregnancy rates.

• Royal Jelly

• Omega-E fatty acid

• New research has shown that melatonin can improve egg quality. Consider taking a melatonin supplement, because new research has shown that the hormone melatonin may help improve egg quality.

• Vitamin B

• DHEA

• Spirulina

• Red raspberry leaf

• Flaxseed

• Coconut oil

• Olive oil

• Grapeseed extract

• Pomegranate

• Kelp

- Bee pollen

- Improve the blood flow and oxygenation to your ovaries. Oxygen rich blood flow to the ovaries is essential for good egg health.
A lack of good blood flow can be due to lack of exercise, dehydration and thick blood. To increase blood flow to the ovaries, drink at least 8 glasses of pure, high-quality water each day. Make sure the water is NOT bottled in plastic. Do light exercise, such as walking. Massage your uterus and ovaries. You might want to look for a massage therapist experienced in abdomen massage

- Hormonal balance is key to proper egg health and cleansing your system of excess hormones can help. You can do this by doing a liver cleanse, especially if you suffer from an overabundance of estrogen.

- Work on improving your uterine health. Some herbs that can help include Burdock Root, Milk Thistle Seed, Dandelion Root, Yellow Dock Root, Licorice Root and Goldenseal Root to cleanse the uterus.

- If your FSH levels are high, consider Vitex, a shrub native to Greece and Italy whose berries have been used in herbal medicine for centuries. Vitex has an amazing ability to balance fertility hormones and is considered one of the most useful herbs in fertility. It helps support and regulate the pituitary gland, inhibits follicle-stimulating hormones, lengthens the luteal phase, and increases progesterone levels.

- Reduce stress as much as you can in your life.

- In Chinese medicine, ovarian health is linked to kidney health. Do a kidney cleanse and eat foods that support and strengthen your kidney.

- Start acupuncture treatments once, twice or three times a week.

- Be aware of the two most common allergens that can impact your body, gluten and dairy.

- Avoid environmental contaminants.

- Avoid dietary fats.

• Be aware of insulin levels and eat in a way that reduces blood sugar level spikes.

• Avoid white flour products

• Repeat affirmations like "my eggs are healthy and can create a beautiful baby."

## • Foods and Substances To Avoid

To maximize your egg health, you want to reduce your exposure to xenohormones, which are substances not found in nature that have hormonal effects on the body. These toxic substances can be absorbed through the skin and build up in the body over time. Sources of xenohormones include solvents and adhesives, including paint, varnish, nail polish and in dry cleaning, car exhaust, all plastics, meat from non-organic livestock, pesticides, herbicides and fungicides, emulsifiers in soap and cosmetics, bug sprays, lawn sprays, and pesticides.

Avoid cosmetics and soaps made with petrochemical emulsifiers.

Do not use mineral oil on your body. Do not microwave your food in plastic. Stop wearing polyester clothing.

• Do not use air fresheners, fabric softeners, spermicide, feminine care products.

• Avoid cigarettes, coffee, alcohol, sugar, non-organic meats and dairy products

• Avoid soda

• Avoid diet foods, processed foods, trans fats and GMO foods.

• Do not eat corn

• Very little to no gluten if possible

- No soy

- Avoid all monounsaturated fats

## • Foods To Enhance Your Egg Health and Quality

- Broccoli, berries, dark leafy vegetables, salmon, pumpkin seeds

- Sesame seeds

- Turmeric

- Dark green leafy vegetables, such as kale, spinach or chard

- Start making your own super fertility smoothie, with ingredients like spinach, strawberries, spirulina, Maca Root, bee pollen, royal jelly, and flax seed.

**Excerpt from Dancing Your Way to Fertility, available on Amazon.com.**

# Strengthening and Preparing Your Organs

As you prepare to be pregnant, it is important to strengthen the various organs in your body.

## • Your Vagina

You want to make your vagina a welcoming environment. A healthy vagina produces healthy cervical mucus, a key to conception. Healthy bacteria in one's vagina can enhance fertility, while an acidic or unhealthy vagina can be a barrier to fertility. Medications, illness, excessive douching, severe emotional stress, or clothing that holds in body heat and moisture, can upset the balance of a healthy vagina. You want to help make your vagina a welcoming environment.

Here are some ways to promote a healthy vagina:

• Wear cotton underwear for good air flow. This prevents the development of damp conditions that promote yeast and unhealthy bacteria. Avoid underwear made from synthetic fabrics, silk, lace and other materials that don't breath freely.

• Do not use douches or feminine sprays that can wash out healthy bacteria that helps the vagina stay clean and infection-free. Avoid scented creams, scented pads, scented tampons and wipes.

• Go to a doctor to see if you have bacterial vaginosis, which is an overgrowth of bacteria inside your vagina and should be treated.

• Check to see if you have any vaginal abnormalities that can impact fertility, such as fusion of the labia or an imperforate hymen.

• It is important not to ignore yeast infections and vaginal infections, such as vulvovaginitis.

• Sexually transmitted diseases, such as Chlamydia and gonorrohea, need to be treated.

• When you wash your vagina, use hot water rather than strong soaps. If you choose to use soap, make sure you thoroughly rinse your vaginal area with warm water so no trace of soap is left behind. Using harsh soaps can lead to infection, and irritation.

• Eat garlic. It has properties that kill yeast.

• Do not use lubricants of any kind.

• Aim to make your vagina less acidic and more sperm friendly. Ideally, your pH range should be at 6.5 to 7.5. If your body is acidic, your cervical mucus will also be acidic, thus creating a hostile environment for sperm.

• Avoid vegetable oil.

• Avoid saliva.

• Avoid glycerin.

• Minimize your intake of sugar, alcohol and white flour products.

• The gut flora, or bacteria in your gut, colonize your vagina. Eat sufficient probiotics or yogurt with bifidus and acidophilus cultures. Yogurt has lactobacillus acidophilus, or "good bacteria." Avoid sugary yogurt.


• L-Arginine increase production of mucus during ovulation.

• Calcium helps the pH balance of the cervical mucus be less acidic and more sperm friendly.

• Grapeseed extract protects the sperm and helpsthe cervical mucus sperm be more sperm-friendly.

• Vitamin C increases the amount of water in your cervical mucus, thus helping produce more cervical mucus.

• Avoid foods that make your blood acidic, such as processed foods, red meat and hydrogenated oils.

• Evening Primrose Oil helps increase cervical mucus production.

• Red clover and Siberian ginseng also help support vaginal health.


## • Ovaries

The ovaries rely on fat for fertility and hormonal balance. Vitamins A and E found in foods such as olive oil and avocados support reproductive health. The antioxidants found in fruits and vegetables, especially those with a deep orange color, are known to strengthen the ovaries. These include sweet potatoes, cantaloupe, oranges, orange bell peppers. Vitamin B6 is also important to ovarian health. If you are deficient in B6, your body may produce more estrogen than you need, which disrupts the menstrual cycle and can prevent your ovaries from releasing eggs on a consistent basis. Foods rich in Vitamin B6 include avocado, spinach, broccoli, beans and potatoes.

# • Thyroid

Undiagnosed thyroid problems can sometimes be at the root cause of infertility or recurrent miscarriages. To start, visit your primary care doctor and have your thyroid tested to find out the amount of the thyroid hormone your thyroid is secreting. Request a thyroid stimulating hormone test (TSH) with the full panel of thyroid levels, including thyroid antibodies and thyroxine. Ask for the numerical result for the TSH level. Some doctors believe that if a woman has a TSH level higher than 2.0, it may indicate that she will have problems getting pregnant.

Hypothyroidism, or an underactive thyroid, and hyperthyroidism, known as over-active thyroid, are sometimes pinpointed as the cause of infertility.

Both hypothyroidism and hyperthyroidism can cause imbalances which impact your ovaries. The ovaries are very sensitive to changes in thyroid levels and even seemingly small declines in thyroid levels can adversely impact ovarian function. Some symptoms of a thyroid dysfunction include cold hands and feet, weight gain and depression.

If you have an underactive thyroid, it means your thyroid gland doesn't produce enough of certain hormones. Low levels of thyroid hormones can interfere with the release of eggs from your ovaries.

That's because the hypothalamus and pituitary glands can sometimes sense an underactive thyroid gland and try to kick things back to normal by increasing the levels of hormones in the body.
 Low levels of the thyroid hormone can interfere with ovulation, which impairs fertility.

Along with being treated by a doctor who specializes in thyroid problems, here are some other things you can do to help your thyroid condition:

• Eat foods high in vitamin A, such as yellow vegetables and dark green vegetables.

• Foods that contain iodine nurture the thyroid, such as kelp and seaweed. Seaweed can be added to soups, salads or just eaten plain. Other foods rich in iodine include: asparagus, bananas, carrots, garlic, onions, spinach, and tomatoes.

• Coconut oil is known to be excellent for boosting thyroid function.

• Foods rich in zinc nourish the thyroid, such as oatmeal, chicken and spinach.

• Raisins are rich in copper, which help the body produce thyroid hormones.

• Soy should not be eaten at this time, because soy can interfere with thyroid hormones.

• The amino acid Tyrosine, found in beef and chicken, help support the thyroid.

• Beet tops, leafy greens, and parsley are helpful in supporting thyroid function.

• Dark green leafy vegetables that are rich in minerals also boost the thyroid.

• Foods to avoid include cauliflower, brussel sprouts, canola oil, soy, peanuts, cabbage and kale, which have goitrogens that are high in sulfur have been known to impede thyroid gland function. A note of caution here, however, those with an overactive thyroid may find these foods helpful. It is recommended you meet with a physician or nutritionist to discuss which foods are best for you, depending on your thyroid condition.

• Avoid coffee, caffeine products and excessive amounts of alcohol.

• Keep your blood sugar levels steady, as fluctuating blood sugar levels can negatively impact the thyroid.

• Avoid artificial sweeteners, such as aspartame.

• Include a good quality sea salt or Celtic salt in your diet, instead of white table salt.

• For an underactive thyroid, consider foods like sea kelp, chicken, dates, molasses, and parsley.

• Reduce your intake of sugar as much as you can.

• Alternative therapies that can help the thyroid include acupuncture and lymph drainage massage, in which the thyroid and lymphatic system are massaged so as to loosen any blocks.

• Avoid drinking out of plastic and soda cans. Instead, drink only out of glass, stainless steel or BPA free plastic bottles.

• Include lots of natural fats in your diet, such as olive oil, flaxseed and avocados.

Vitamin and mineral supplements considered helpful to thyroid function include:

• B-complex

• Vitamin C

• Omega 3s that are found in fish, flaxseed and walnuts, which are the building blocks for the hormones that control immune function and cell growth.

• A multi-mineral formula in liquid form, since minerals are key to glandular health.

• Calcium/magnesium are also known to help the metabolic process.

• High-quality natural thyroid supplements. Note: you may want to seek the advice of a well-trained nutritionist on what type of supplements are appropriate for those who are trying to get pregnant, and what dosage is appropriate once you are pregnant or on infertility medications.

• You might want to consider a glutathione supplement and include in your diet foods that contain glutathione, such as asparagus, broccoli, peaches, spinach, garlic and grapefruit.

• Pay attention to your food allergies and sensitivies.

• Reduce gluten in your diet or if you can, go entirely gluten free.

• Take a probiotic, because for the thyroid to be healthy and function well, it needs and depends on having a sufficient supply of healthy gut bacteria.

• Pay attention to adrenal burn-out or fatigue, because there is a strong connection between the thyroid and adrenal glands. Think of the thyroid and adrenals as Frick and Frack—if you have a problem with hypothyroidism, you are probably suffering with some level of adrenal fatigue or burn-out too.

• Include seaweed in your diet.

• Avoid excessive forms of radiation if you can.

• Do a heavy metal cleanse. Heavy metal exposure is sometimes linked to thyroid problems. In addition to a heavy metal cleanse, begin eating or juicing garlic and cilantro, and include such as taking Milk Thistle, turmeric and chlorella in your diet.

• Eat more foods that contain selenium, such as salmon, sunflower seeds, onions and brazil nuts.

• Stress and emotional traumas, such as a job loss or marital problems, can weaken thyroid function. Explore creative ways to reduce stress, such as joining a chorus, taking gentle walks in a beautiful area, or take a painting or drawing class. Deep breath.

• The thyroid gland is located in the throat, the center of our communication with the world. Holistic practitioners often view low thyroid function as a result of a blocked throat chakra, a result of feeling like you can't speak your truth. It is important to learn new and creative ways of finding and using your voice, such as singing, writing and creating art. Stop 'swallowing' your feelings. Speak your truth instead. Create an expression center in your home, where you feel safe to freely say what you want to say and let your deepest feelings be known.

• Avoid drinking tap water.

• Do not use non-stick cookware.

• Stop using perfume for now, especially in the neck area.

• Eat foods that contain tyrosine, an amino acid the body needs to manufacture thyroid hormones, such as avocados, almonds, bananas, pumpkin seeds and lentils.

• Include more sea vegetables in your diet, such as kelp and kelp granules that can be sprinkled over your salads.

• Stay outside in the sunshine at least 20 minutes a day.

• Evening primrose oil is rich in amino acids which nourish the thyroid gland.

• Consider taking the herbs Nettle and Bladder Wrack.

• Discontinue using deodorants and body lotions that contain parabens, chlorates and pesticides.

## • Your Spleen and Digestive System

The spleen is an important organ involved in the hormonal cycle and is responsible for certain types of progesterone production. It also governs many of the energetic processes in the body. Balancing your digestive system and spleen can help you achieve the right balance of floras in your system to increase your fertility.

The spleen also impacts the thyroid hormone and progesterone production. Some link menstrual difficulties to a spleen imbalance.

Some ways to strengthen and balance your spleen and digestive system include:

• In Chinese medicine, the emotion associated with the Spleen is worry. It is important for spleen health to learn to say no without reason or excuse and make a concerted effort to take care of yourself each day.

• Consider digestive enzymes, with hydrochloric acid, available at health food stores.

• Consider probiotics to increase 'good gut bacteria.'

• Avoid sodas and drink lots of water instead. Lack of water is sometimes the cause of poor digestion.

• Chew your food slowly

• Include ground flaxseed in your diet.

• Increase fiber in your diet, with foods like apples, figs, prunes and dates.

• Acupuncture has been reported to encourage healthy digestion.

• Avoid sugar, white flour products, raw cold foods, soy and dairy products.

• Try to walk each day. Exercise helps move the spleen energy.

• Eliminate possible food allergens in your diet.

• Boost friendly bacteria in your body.

• Massage your stomach to help reduce stress and aid digestion.

# • Pituitary Gland

The pituitary gland is sometimes called the master gland of the body, because all the other endocrine glands depend on its secretion for stimulation. It is a tiny gland located at the base of the brain and is sometimes referred to as the thermostat of the body because it controls the other hormone secreting glands. High protein foods help the pituitary gland release its hormones, because the building blocks of proteins are amino acids.

Emotionally, problems with the pituitary gland can come from not respecting your inner wisdom and/or pretending to be someone your not.

Supplements that can help the pituitary gland include:

• Bee pollen

• Spirulina

• Magnesium

• Potassium

• Dandelion

• Omega-3 oil

• Chia seeds

Other ways to help the pituitary gland include:

• Manganese is important to a healthy pituitary gland. Foods that contain manganese include citrus fruits, greens and egg yokes.

• Walk at least 20 minutes a day in sunlight. This will encourage the pituitary gland to produce helpful levels of ovary-stimulating hormones. You also might want to consider a Vitamin D supplement.

• L-Arginine is an amino acid that promotes the section of HGH.

• Fenugreek stimulates the release of HGH while giving your energy levels a kick.

• Get more sleep

• In traditional Chinese medicine, the emotional aspect of pituitary gland health involves bonding with others, sharing words and ideals. Think about and journal about this aspect of your life. Do you feel you are adequately and healthily bonding with others? Are there people in your life where you can take down your 'walls' and share your words and ideals?

• Include meat and protein in your diet.

## • Hypothalamus and thymus

The hypothalamus regulates the pituitary gland and secretes hormones that control the thyroid, adrenals, ovaries and testes.

Here are some ways to support your hypothalamus:

• A handful of sunflower seeds each day can boost the hypothalamus. Sunflower seeds contain B1 or thiamine, which is crucial for hypothalamus health.

• Eat foods rich in Vitamin C, including red bell peppers, oranges, lemons.

• Seaweed

• Pumpkin seeds

# • Pineal Gland

The pineal gland controls the circadian rhythms in the body, as well as melatonin and pinoline production.

The pineal gland manufactures melatonin, a hormone that plays a key role in fertility, because it controls the timing and release of many key reproductive hormones. In Chinese medicine melatonin is linked to healthy liver energy, considered very important to reproductive health. Having adequate amounts of melatonin in your body has been shown to improve pregnancy rates. Because we live in a light-saturated culture due to TVs, cell phones, computer screens and street lights, we are often robbed of the melatonin we need for a restful night's sleep. Sleep disturbances are a recipe for hormonal imbalance.

Here are some ways to strengthen the pineal gland:

• Fluoride is the number one enemy of a healthy pineal gland. The mineral boron, found in beets and dried plums, can help remove fluoride from the human body.

• Coffee, alcohol and tobacco weaken the pineal gland.

• Apple cider vinegar strengthens the pineal gland.

• Oregano and garlic are considered helpful to pineal gland health.

• Consider a Melatonin supplement.

• Sunlight acts as a food for the pineal gland

• Chlorophyll-rich superfoods, like spirulina and chlorella, detoxify the pineal gland

• Add natural food sources of iodine to your diet, such as seaweed

• Foods that strengthen the pineal gland include watermelon, coconut oil, spinach, asparagus and broccoli.

# • Pancreas

Keeping your pancreas healthy and your blood sugar levels stable will help stabilize your hormones when you are trying to get pregnant. When blood sugar levels are high, we suffer spikes that weaken our adrenal glands. Sugar frazzles the hormones and leaves our endocrine system exhausted. When our sugar levels drop, our adrenals release both cortisol and adrenaline in an attempt to restore our sugar levels back to an even kneel, leading to hormonal imbalance.

The reason these sugar spikes impact our fertility is that progesterone, which is the main hormone required for ovulation, and cortisol compete for the same receptor binding sites in the body. Cortisol, however, will always win this showdown. When these hormones battle, it disrupts the entire endocrine system, which in turn, disrupts all the sex hormones, including oestrogen, progesterone, and the androgen DHEA.

To keep your hormones in tip-top shape, reduce your sugar intake.

Here are some ways to keep your pancreas healthy and your blood sugar levels stable:

• Eat foods that nourish your pancreas, such as blueberries, sunflower seeds, almonds, cherries, broccoli, garlic, red grapes, spinach, sweet potatoes. Prepare these foods ahead of time and carry them with you so you can have them available wherever you go.

• Eat something healthy every three hours.

• Eat lots of spinach, which is high in magnesium and is known to help prevent type 2 diabetes.

• Avocados are also high in magnesium.

- Walnuts, which are high in monounsaturated fat, help stabilize blood sugar levels.

- Get at least eight hours of sleep.

- Almonds can lessen the subsequent rise in blood sugar.

- Avoid soda and artificial sweeteners.

**A Bonus Excerpt from Dancing Your Way to Fertility, available on Amazon.com.**

**My doctor looked at me point blank and said without a trace of mercy that my eggs were "bottom of the barrel."**

**Bottom of the barrel... Her words rang in my head like a cruel pronouncement.**

**I was 37 years old and desperately wanted a second child. My doctor didn't believe I could have one.**

**I had been through this before. To have my daughter, I endured 10 IUIs, several operations and too many nights of crying to count.**

**So I left her office: desperate, heartbroken, and wildly, frantically panicked. The words 'your eggs are bottom of the barrel' kept repeating in my head. Despite everything I've gone through, I always had hope. My insides were screaming: 'I can't live with this.' I was so shaken, I could barely drive home. Her words nearly broke my will and spirit to try again.**

**For some reason, on the way home, I stopped at a natural foods market. Walking around the supermarket, amidst all the healthy foods and supplements, I began to question what the doctor told me. Was the poor quality of my eggs something that could be improved? Was I unhealthy on some undetectable level that was impacting my fertility?**

I went home and called my ever-wise mother. She gave me great advice: dump that doctor and try again.

I did exactly what Mom said.

I decided I would do everything I could to restore and heal my fertility, and not be hindered by my age, regardless of what the doctor said.

Over time, I learned that there was hope for me and others like me—and just because a doctor says you can never get pregnant does not mean your body, if given the right elements, cannot heal from infertility.

My devastation and despair turned to determination, and everything I learned, I put in this book. As a newspaper reporter for more than 25 years, I utilized my skills as a journalist to get to the root of fertility problems, the physical and the emotional.

I am now also a fertility success certified life coach.

I wrote this book for those of you suffering with infertility, who like me who have been told that your eggs are too old, that your body is too unhealthy, weak, or damaged, that there is little hope.

I wrote this book for all of you who feel that having a child is some type of impossible dream, that you are the victim of some pathologically cruel biological problem.

I wrote it for you brave survivors of infertility who dream of starting a family, but find the road long, cruel, uphill, and not always forgiving of slight mistakes and accumulated years.

Together, we will work to heal everything in your body and mind that could be stopping you from getting pregnant. Consider me your personal fertility success coach.

I will help you identify all the physical and emotional obstacles that might be standing in the way of your having the children you desire. Then-one-by-one, we are going to knock these obstacles out of your body and your life.

I created the Ultimate Fertility Success Program, which I believe is one of the most comprehensive body-mind makeover plans available to fertility patients today.

The Ultimate Fertility Success Program includes 12 cleanses that will detoxify your body and expand your fertility potential. It will also show you how to improve the quality of your eggs—something previously not thought possible—and balance your hormones.

It includes a chapter on strengthening, preparing, and emotionally and spiritually healing every organ in your body that impacts your fertility.

Then we will look at the foods you eat, the lifestyle you live, and vitamins and herbs that will give you a fair and fighting chance to enjoy vibrant fertility. You may be eating, thinking and experiencing life in a way that is depleting your reproductive organs, and you didn't even know it.

The program is designed to change the track you are on so you can become more healthy, vibrant and fertile—as you deserve to be!

For your guy, I've included The Ultimate Male Fertility Preparation Plan, that includes little known information to help your guy enhance his fertility.

We will address all the obvious and not so obvious blocks to your fertility, because some fertility problems are difficult to diagnose and there are not yet diagnostic tools available to detect the slight shifts, blocks, and traumas in the body that can prevent or delay pregnancy. The traumas and painful emotions we experience can lodge themselves in our cells, interrupting our body's natural healthy energy flow.

This book will help you examine all aspects of your life, from your childhood and family experiences, to your deepest thoughts and beliefs about pregnancy and motherhood, so that you are fully aware of your subconscious feelings and beliefs and every part of you can work together to have the babies of your dreams.

I will share with you the information you need to unblock and destroy the emotional and spiritual traumas, thoughts and fears that could secretly be preventing your body from having a baby.

I've included 50 art, writing, music and dance activities you can do in your home to help you unlock your creative reproductive powers and release negative energy patterns in your body.

Everything in this book can be used in conjunction with an IVF, IUI or other assisted reproductive technologies. We will discuss how to prepare for an IUI and/or IVF, and how to treat yourself the days following these procedures to maximize your chances of getting pregnant.

I have included my own story of battling infertility that I hope you will find useful and inspiring.

As a bonus, I'm including:

• Your Fertility Food Tracker Diary: Its simple, easy to use and will help you track what fertility foods you are giving your body each day.

I've also included several other free journals. These include:

• Journal Writing Through Your Subconscious: to help you discover what your deepest consciousness truly thinks about fertility, motherhood and parenting.

• Your Daily Happiness Journal: to help you gain access to your inner positive-feeling antenna that is ever alert to everything good within you and around you.

• Life Affirmation Journal: designed to help you take note of all the ways birth and life take place in the world around you each day, and how you are intrinsically part of the world's never-ending reproductive cycle.

• My Child & I Journal: where you can share your dreams of a future with your children by your side.

• Emotional Tracking Journal: to help you understand what triggers your positive and negative emotions each day.

This book will also discuss how to:

• Deal with negative comments from friends and relatives, as well as your own internal negativity.

• How to not let infertility ruin your marriage.

• How to choose the right doctor and clinic.

• Ways to reduce stress in your life.

• Writing exercises that will give you a chance to go deep within to unearth and destroy all the self-defeating beliefs and traumas that might be buried deep in your tissues that could be destroying your fertility.

• More than 100 affirmations and visualizations.

• A personal fertility vision statement, that I have written as a certified life coach. It is used to help motivate and get you past the blocks and obstacles to your fertility. You can listen to and read it each day.

• Letters you can send yourself, or just leave around the house, when you need a lift or a reminder of how strong and powerful you really are.

- How to start enjoying a close loving friendship with your body, so your body becomes your best friend and teammate.

- How to turn your home into a fertility nesting center.

- Coping with the unfairness of it all.

- Ways to protect your baby once you are pregnant

And all my mistakes (which were many) you can learn from.

This is, most importantly, a book of hope…and about taking action to have the children you deserve and are worthy of.

That doctor who claimed my eggs were 'bottom of the barrel' was wrong. Less than a year later, I gave birth to my beautiful son.

Someday, I would like to send her a picture of my boy and write in blazing letters across the picture: "Is this what bottom of the barrel looks like?"

Extra Bonus Excerpt from Dancing Your Way to Fertility available on Amazon.com or at www.dancingyourwaytofertility.com

## Infertility: A Training Ground for Motherhood?

In times past, women have always endured sacrifice and trial as part of motherhood. Now, due to a host of factors such as age, health and environment, women are put through a severe test of their maternal stamina even before they conceive their child.

This road, this test, this initiation, will test all of you--and it will make you one of the strongest, most capable, confident, resourceful, perseverant mothers a child could ever have. Experiencing infertility gives you a lifetime pass to enjoy motherhood in a way few ever get to enjoy it, because with the difficulties of this disease come confidence and appreciation.

This journey will demand all the best parts of you. It will demand you persevere when you want to give up. It will demand patience and persistence when frustration and helpless surrender might feel like a more natural path.

It will demand that every survival skill you possess be brought forth and utilized. It will demand sacrifice, self-preservation, and a willpower beyond what you knew you had, but what intrinsically you knew you were capable of.

If you are not fortunate, you may have your heart broken in 1000 pieces.

If you are fortunate, you could still have your heart broken in 1000 places.

When you give birth to your baby none of it will matter. Your heart will heal, the scars will seem insignificant, and all the tears, disappointments and devastations will seem like bunny rabbits and balloons on a summer's day.

No big deal.

If you do not give birth to a baby, but decide to adopt, become a foster parent, a teacher, coach, counselor or play a very active role in the life of a young niece, nephew, neighbor, or cousin, you will be ready and able to mother these children and impact a younger generation in a way more powerful than you ever imagined.

You have probably been through the best training course for motherhood possible: you understand pain, you understand the potential for joy, you are willing to do the work to get the child you want, and you've proven you can take the bad stuff that comes with going after the good stuff. In doing this, you will join a group of super cultivated mothers, women ready to nurture and love the next generation, and have more than proven their worth to do this.

Infertility hurts.

Winning over infertility can be a painful process that demands resolve and sacrifice.

It is an initiation rite, of sorts, an involuntary one, of course.

No one should have to go through this to have a baby and no one would voluntarily choose this road. Nonetheless, it is a reality for many of us, and it will prepare you for motherhood in a grand and inspiring way that someday you may even feel thankful to have experienced.

It is a long road and an unfair one, but at the end of the road, you could be holding the baby of your dreams, just as the same as someone who made love one night and woke up pregnant the next morning.

Then nothing at all will matter but your baby.